CW00495566

# Remember to grab your free bonus!

Go to: www.JuicetoLoseWeight.com now to download

- 26 Pro-Tasting Juices for Weight Loss Recipes
- Learn the 1 SECRET on losing weight that NOBODY talks about
- Weight loss hack to avoid hitting a plateau
- Plus more weight loss hacks and support via email!

# Table of Contents

# Introduction

Before you read on, know that this book is unlike many other juicing books out there. The information I share is a real life tried and tested method I personally use to lose 20 pounds to date. The tips I share are not only practical, but also effective in keeping the weight loss off for good.

Losing weight has been a constant struggle for me, since my teens. Back then, I wasn't overweight because of the physical activities I often engaged in. However, the lack of education in diet, and taking my high metabolism rate for granted soon surfaced on the weighing scale as I got older. My activity level declined because I was just too busy with high school and college (read: lazy and tired).

I was still doing okay at this point, because I played tennis and had friends who were running enthusiasts and dragged me along to train for mini-marathons. Still, I took my diet for granted, thinking that I would simply burn off whatever I ate.

However, all these changed when I had kids. I was too busy to even look after myself. I ate out a lot because I didn't have time to cook healthily for myself. Breastfeeding kept my weight somewhat in check, but still the problem was there - I wasn't eating as well as I should.

The wake-up call came to me when I weighed in at 141 pounds.

I had never been this heavy, even after pregnancy. Reality sank in. I could no longer fit into my regular clothes and became upset when shop assistants handed me size 14 clothes. Pictures of myself highlighted my flabby arms and belly that I couldn't suck in anymore.

My husband, who had always said little about how I looked, finally commented, "I think it's time you really watch your diet and lose some weight."

I took up exercise programmes like Insanity Workout and P90x which took up way too much time, before settling with Focus T25 that only took up 30 minutes each day for me and had modified moves to help me feel less lousy about my fitness level.

Still, they didn't help me to lose weight. I just got heavier and heavier.

I guess deep down inside my heart, I knew what I needed to do. I had to start eating better if I wanted to see any dip in my weight. My usual diet consisted of less than 10% vegetables, and I knew that this was the problem. I was consuming way too much carbs, and being gluten sensitive, the problem was quite obvious.

But, I hated the way vegetables tasted. I tried to cook them at home but they didn't seem to taste good without adding extra salt and seasonings. I dreaded the bland tastes of vegetables and it didn't took more than a day for me to give up and head back to my old diet that was making me fatter and unhealthier.

I knew I had to do something about it, and that was when I chanced upon Juicing.

I thought, hey I could drink down a salad instead of eat it.

A quick Google search for simple recipes and guidelines, and the rest is pretty much history. I was steadily dropping 2 pounds a week!

At the time of writing this book, I am down to 120 pounds. Not my ideal weight yet, but I can foresee myself hitting my target weight in a matter of a few months.

I have finally found something that works for me, that involves a lifestyle change for me which I can sustain in the long run. I've become more conscious about my food choices, and my taste buds are more sensitive and receptive to what used to be bland-tasting vegetables. I now enjoy my juices at least once a day, and give myself a pampering treat with a cheat day over the weekend. (And still maintaining my weight loss!)

IBS has become non-existent for me, and I have never felt much better and LIGHTER than before. In fact now at the age of 27, I feel much healthier than I was at 17!

If like me, you have been struggling with eating greens, trying to ditch the weight and embrace healthier eating habits, then this book is definitely the answer to your weight loss prayers.

In this book, we will explore the reasons of unsuccessful weight loss (despite doing everything right), why Juicing for weight loss is an effective solution long-term weight loss, and my 4-week juicing plan that is sure to bring you results.

The recipes I share are simple to put together, TASTY and easy to follow.

However, this book will NOT cover juice cleanses if this is what you are looking for. Because I have personally attempted juice cleanses and they bring no more results that the 4-week juicing plan I devised for myself (and I will explain why in another chapter).

By the way, I have also not gone back to any of the exercise programmes, simply because I wanted to prove to myself and to friends that weight loss is contributed by 70-80% nutrition, more than exercise. I'm sure this sounds really good, because you no longer have to put in hours of training a week to lose weight, especially if you are a busy parent like me!

So if you are ready to ditch the weight, and give yourself an achievable head start in eating healthily, read on and be ready to welcome the new you!

## Why Are You Still Not Losing Weight?

The problem with fad diets and fad workout programs is that while they have been proven to be effective, most of us just can't seem to keep them part of our lifestyle for very long.

Nutrition experts say that sticking to rigid diet or workout plans are difficult to maintain over the long-term. Sure, they are very effective in helping people to lose weight, but guess what happens after you've gotten your results? That's right, you put back all the weight, or worse, you become heavier than before!

Would I consider Juicing a "fad diet?" Not so much as long as you make it part of your lifestyle, which is why I wrote this book. If you consider Juicing to be just a quick-fix for you, or think you could get away with doing a Juice cleanse, then you should reconsider your weight loss goal.

Besides, losing weight also involves determination and a conscious effort to make decisions that will benefit your body. So if you have had some success with a fad diet or exercise program and are still reading this book anyway, I believe that you are looking for something that produces more permanent results.

Besides the rigidity of most fad diet plans, here are some other reasons why you're still not losing weight:

**Not Eating Right**

You think you are eating healthy because you eat "low-carb" meal replacements and sugar-free snacks but these products often contain preservatives and highly processed ingredients. If you are eating low-carb products that come in a box, are wrapped or packaged, then you probably should not be eating them. You should eat real food, not processed products. You can eat avocados but think twice before you buy that guacamole from the grocery store.

You may also be watching your calorie intake, but the quality of calories also differ in foods. 100 calories in a can of soda isn't the same as 100 calories in a plate of greens. So while you do count your calories, watch what you eat as well.

**Not Engaging in Enjoyable Physical Activity**

I love doing sprints and I hate running long distances. I used to force myself to go on long runs, thinking that the longer I ran, the more I would be exercising, but I was so wrong. I got so frustrated my muscles tensed up every time I went for a run. And obviously, I didn't stick to that habit for very long because I hated running.

Then a friend introduced me to doing intermittent sprinting, and I loved it! I got the results I wanted, decided to engage in other activities I enjoyed doing and felt so much better. Finding an activity you like also ensures that you are more likely to stick to the routine

So the next time your friend recommends you something new because it worked for him/her, think twice about it. Sign up for trial classes and see whether you like it. Just because your friend has lost 5 pounds by running on the treadmill for an hour everyday, doesn't mean you are going to get the same results too.

**Not Getting Enough Veggies**

This is very close to heart because I found myself having problems to lose weight because I simply dreaded the taste of vegetables. After I got into Juicing, I was able to increase my intake of vegetables. Weight loss was a result of this change, and my digestive problems seem to have been resolved!

**Not Equating Weight Loss to Lifestyle Change**

A change in lifestyle is the key to weight loss, not diets. There are diets which may help you lose weight but most diets are so restrictive, they can be unhealthy in the long run. Rather than go on a diet, get back to basics and focus on your overall health. What you need is a change in lifestyle, a lifestyle that includes good nutrition, exercise, and a balance among the different aspects of your life. Make smart choices and try to get the most nutrition for the calories you consume.

When your food choices and physical activities become a part of your lifestyle that you can maintain, that's when weight loss becomes an almost natural benefit that follows.

Also as I mentioned earlier, the goal is to lose the weight permanently. So in order to achieve the weight loss results you want, you need to set your mind on developing healthy lifestyle habits that enable you to get long-term health benefits.

Which is why I devised my 4-Week Juicing for Weight Loss plan to help you ease into the Juicing lifestyle, and make sure it is a sustainable diet for you.

## Should You Do a Juice Cleanse?

Many juicers advocate doing a Juice Cleanse before you start your new diet plan or exercise regime. The purpose is to detox, cleanse or "spring clean" your system, getting rid of all the accumulated junk in your system. This way, when you begin a new diet plan, your body will be able to absorb the nutrients much better without the junk blocking up the absorption.

**The benefits of a Juice Cleanse/Fast is as follows:**

- Rest your stomach
- Rest and repair your gut
- Rest your liver
- Reduces your appetite
- Ease food decision-making
- Eliminate harmful foods
- Flood your body with super nutrition
- Lose weight

- Improve energy
- Rehydrate your odd
- Reduce physical problems
- Allow maximum detoxification

(Source: HuffingtonPost "The Real Reasons Juice Cleanses Can Get Your Health Back on Track")

I personally recommend doing a Juice Cleanse occasionally, BUT **I do not recommend** doing one if you are just starting to Juice. This is because of the potential side effects that I believe would steer you away for even wanting to incorporate Juicing in your lifestyle, such as:

From a personal perspective, I can honestly tell you a Juice Cleanse SUCKS. I felt sleepy, grumpy, had migraines and couldn't concentrate at all. Unless you can take a couple of days off and not give a care about the world, the potential side effects of a Juice Cleanse can make you experience:

- Menstrual cycle changes
- Bowel movements that smell foul
- Sinus
- Extreme nausea and maybe vomiting
- Bad breathe
- Worsening body door
- Skin worsens

You may also experience ailments you used to have such as colds, fevers, skin spots, headaches, pimples, fatigue, dizziness, runny nose and low energy. All these side effects are believed to be part of the body purging all the toxins, which makes sense. Also, doing a Juice Cleanse involves a sudden dip in calorie intake, which could account for the decrease in energy level (Source: All About Juicing).

Now I know that there are people who do Juice Cleanses for more than a week and have mentioned that it feels better after the first couple of days. In fact, they felt like a brand new person after the Juice

Cleanse and congratulate themselves for having won the "mental game." Personally, I felt horrible during the first couple of days of my Juice cleanse, to the point of wanting to give up. This can be a bad thing because it would potentially make you drop the idea of Juicing, thinking it is just another fad diet that your weak willpower cannot overcome. (Yes, I have a weak willpower when it comes to doing a Juice Cleanse, but I still managed to lose weight, didn't I?)

And this is what we want to avoid!

I am also a believer that once you start to gradually introduce juice into your diet and start to drink more water, your body knows what it needs to do and will clean itself out eventually. That's what your liver, kidneys and intestines are for! In fact, Dr John Emsley was quoted in the Washington Times as saying that "our bodies are very good at eliminating all the nasties that we might ingest over the festive season."

In fact, most of the weight you lose in a Juice Cleanse is more likely water weight, which will be put back soon after you go back to your normal diet and start eating solid foods. I say this with certainty also because I have attempted a 3 day Juice Cleanse, lost 10 pounds and put back 8 pounds the following week. This gave me a net loss of 2 pounds, which is EASILY attainable by just incorporating Juicing into your lifestyle, without all the undesirable side effects that challenge your willpower.

So now, even if I see the need to do a Juice Cleanse, 1 or 2 days is more than sufficient for my body to do what it needs to do.

And yes, I welcome cheat days where I indulge and eat whatever I want too!

## How Does Juicing Help You to Lose Weight (for good)?

Juicing means you extract juice from fruits and vegetables rather than eating them whole. Juices are quickly absorbed into the bloodstream and offer immediate benefits. Some people go for juicing to boost their immune system or to clear up a skin condition or disease. But nowadays, juicing is also done to manage weight.

Juicing helps people lose weight. Raw juices are full of antioxidants which bind toxins and carry them out of the body. Since many of these toxins are stored in fat, you can shed weight at a quicker pace.

**Increases intake of nutrients from greens**

If you don't want to eat your fruits and vegetables, don't worry about getting your nutrients because you can drink them. By juicing, you can get all the minerals, vitamins, and enzymes you need to stay healthy.

Juicing helps increase your intake of fresh produce. Vegetables and fruits are important to supply your body with vitamins and minerals that help boost immunity. But most people do not get the recommended amount of vegetables and fruits daily. They find it hard to consume that many vegetables. Fortunately, juicing can get them to quickly consume an equivalent amount of these vegetables.

There are good reasons why you should consider juicing. It allows your body to absorb nutrients faster. It also helps you consume the recommended daily amount of vegetables and allows you to add a variety of vegetables to your diet.

**Juicing as part of a lifestyle**

When it comes to nutrition, it is easy for people with busy schedules and multiple commitments to make poor choices. Juicing can help you live a healthy life and a life full of energy. It can easily be incorporated into your busy life.

Instead of drinking coffee in the morning, substitute it with a glass of fruit juice then perhaps another glass in the afternoon and in the early evening. Within a short period of time, you may start to feel a difference in your health.

You may even begin experimenting with other vegetables and fruits juices. As you enjoy its benefits, it becomes easy to make juicing part of your daily routine and your normal life.

**Suppresses food cravings**

Most of the time, you crave for food because the body is starving for nutrients which are supposed to be in the food that you take. Unfortunately, most of the modern diet lacks the proper nutrients that the body needs, so your body tries to fill the absence of the nutrient by increasing your cravings. Juicing can very well provide these nutrients that the body desperately needs. Therefore, you are going to have less cravings for food.

Fresh vegetable juice works as an appetite suppressant and curbs cravings for food. When you are juicing for weight loss, drink a glass of fresh juice before your main meal to ease your hunger and at the same time provide you with the needed minerals and vitamins.

Juicing supports your weight loss goals by reducing your food cravings, boosting your metabolism, supporting the natural fat burning processes of your body, supplying your cells with nutrients, reducing the acidity in your body, and flushing out the toxins stored in your fat cells.

**Provides more energy**

When drinking fruit and vegetable juices, you are reducing the digestive process that occurs when you consume food. Juicing has removed the fibers from the vegetables and fruits, leaving the nutrients, minerals, vitamins, enzymes, and antioxidants which are easily absorbed into your system and becomes immediately available for use by the body.

Your digestive system does not have to work as hard as when it digests hard meats, heavy bread, and dairy products. You can use the energy that the digestive system would have used, making you feel more active, happy, and healthy.

The bottom line is that juicing can be an effective weight loss program because it can reduce calorie intake and can satiate hunger without sacrificing the minerals and nutrients needed by the body.

## The Great Juicer Debate

Which juicer is best for you? Is a Slow Juicer (aka masticating juicer) the best for you? But what if you only have a Centrifugal, high speed juicer?

**Read: The best juicer is the one you really use.**

See, how simple was that!

Now, let's look at the pros and cons of each juicer...

### The Centrifugal Juicer

A centrifugal juicer is the most common type of juicing machine and is more affordable. It works well with soft and hard vegetables and fruits, but not so well with leafy vegetables such as spinach or kale in extracting the juices out. The centrifugal juicer spins at high speed. This grounds the vegetables or fruits that you push down the chute into a pulp. The same spinning motion separates the juice from the pulp.

The juice that is produced by a centrifugal juicer has more foam because of the high-speed spinning which can trap more air and cause frothing.

Some people say that the high speed action also produces too much heat which may kill the enzymes in the juice. This is why the juice extracted by the centrifugal juicer must be consumed right away.

Most of the centrifugal juicers I've tried out generate quite some of noise, which is most likely due to the spinning of the blades and chopping of the ingredients.  Yet, a centrifugal juicer can easily fit into anyone's budget. And because it operates at high-speed, you get your juice much faster. I can prepare a 32 oz juice in 15 minutes, from cutting up my ingredients to washing up. I usually drink juices prepared from my Philips HR1871 Centrifugal juicer within 30 minutes. If I kept them till more than 12 hours later, there is an obvious change in taste for me.

**The Masticating Juicer**

The masticating juicers are more pricey than the centrifugal models. It works quietly at low speed with no spinning action. The slow crushing and squeezing action is the reason why this masticating juicer can juice soft and leafy green veggies such as spinach, parsley, cilantro, kale, and wheatgrass. Because of its low speed action, it allows you to juice more vegetables with greater efficiency.

The juicer yields at least 20 to 30% more juice compared to the centrifugal juicing machine. You can even save on vegetables because it requires less vegetables to produce more juice.

Its low-speed but powerful motor eliminates oxidation so it can preserve the enzymes and the nutrients of the juices. The juice that the masticating juicer makes has very little foam. It can even reduce the amount of pesticides in the juice that it makes, that is, if you have not used organic vegetables or fruits. Since the juice it makes can last longer, you can make a large batch of juice which you can store for future use.

One big advantage of the masticating juicer is its versatility. It can make baby food, grind coffee beans and spices, mince herbs, and turn nuts into nut butter. I love my Hurom Slow Juicer because it is also very easy to clean up.

**Still Confused? Here's are some factors to help you choose the best juicer for your lifestyle:**

**Budget:** If budget is the most important thing for you right now, get a Centrifugal juicer like the Philips HR1871. When you feel like you are ready to spend more for quality juice, you can eventually upgrade to a masticating juicer.

**Time:** This is a bit tricky to explain because it depends on how your schedule is like. If you are those who prefer to make your juice and finish cleaning up your juicer in 15 minutes, then a Centrifugal juicer is ideal, as long as you consume your juice as soon as possible.

If you prefer to set some time out twice a week and prepare a batch of juices that you can "grab and go," then a masticating juicer is ideal for you.

**Quality:** The slow juicer is definitely your best bet if you are very concerned with juice quality, as heat from the high-spinning Centrifugal juicer would result in some nutrient loss, thereby affecting juice quality.

I personally have both the Centrifugal and Masticating Juicer, although I use the latter much more often these days. I have learnt to set aside a couple of hours each week to buy my groceries and prepare my juices. That's also because I have a very small fridge and it seems more space efficient to juice a batch and store them in jars instead. :)

Although my Hurom Juicer was a hefty investment at the start, it has worked out for me in the long run. I am able to save on vegetables and fruits because it produces more juice from less produce. I like the fact that it can preserve the enzymes and nutrients of the juices. I also enjoy its versatility. Aside from juicing, I have used it to mince herbs and to make peanut butter. I like to work in my kitchen quietly so the masticating juicer is perfect for me because it operates quietly.

## How to Maximize Juice Output

Now that you understand the pros and cons of each juicer, you now need to know how to juice your ingredients to maximise juice output.

### Centrifugal Juicer

I find that the most efficient way of preparing your juice with a centrifugal juicer is to wash and cut up all the ingredients together, as you can run them very quickly through your juicer. If you are using apples, it's a good idea to juice them first, as they tend to oxidise quickly.

It is recommended to "sandwich" your softer ingredients such as leafy greens in between 2 harder ingredients. For example, sandwiching Kale leaves between apple and carrots.

You can also alternate between soft and hard ingredients. The hard ingredients ensure that any remnants of the softer ingredients will be pushed through your juicer.

**Masticating/Slow Juicer**

Well, you understand that running your ingredients through a slow juicer is going to take a much longer time, and lots of patience as compared to using a Centrifugal juicer.

Some Juicers advocate sandwiching the soft ingredients between hard ingredients like how you would do it with a Centrifugal juicer. However, after experimenting with my Hurom juicer and getting tips from the Hurom people, the best way seems to be running the softest ingredients first, followed by the hardest ingredient last.

So in this way, you would be running the leafy greens first and slowly, followed by juicing an apple or carrot last. This really forces all the stuff in the juicer to be pushed out, thereby maximising juice output.

Note that in this way, what's most efficient is to prepare the soft ingredients first, then prepare the rest of the ingredients while the softer ones are being juiced. If you have a slow juicer you would know exactly what I'm talking about when I say you need lots of patience. But that is worth it, for the quality of juice you get!

Also, since apples oxidise very quickly, you can leave them out until they are really needed before cutting them up!

---

Hopefully I have helped you to decide on which is the best Juicer for you. Now, we are ready to hit the stores and grab our ingredients to start juicing!

## The 4-Week Juicing for Weight Loss Plan

Finally! We're going to dive into how to get started to lose weight. If you haven't read the earlier chapters, I totally recommend you do so. They're a quick read and help eliminate any misconceptions and questions you have about the Juicing for Weight Loss plan.

This plan is designed to EASE you into the Juicing lifestyle, week by week. By the end of 4 weeks, you will experience as much as 10 pounds of weight loss, which is what I personally witnessed in my own body, and it isn't water weight at all! I have a good friend who followed my plan, continued to exercise 3 times a week, didn't give herself a single cheat day and managed to ditch 15 pounds.

The amount you are likely to lose will depend on your diet and activity level during this 4 weeks. However, my goal for YOU is to lose 2 pounds over this 4 weeks, which is TOTALLY ACHIEVABLE, don't you think?

So, when you begin on this 4-Week Juicing plan, bear in mind that Juicing will become part of your lifestyle and it will be SO EASY to Juice everyday, that you would feel totally uneasy if you haven't had your daily dose of Juice ;)

**Here are some tips to follow as you embark on your Juicing journey to lose weight:**

- Add an extra fruit if the taste is not palatable enough, then work towards reducing the fruit portion
- Start with a smaller portion of leafy greens and increase until you are used to the taste
- Feel free to play around with different fruits to see which ones you like best (for example, replace oranges with apples)
- Experiment with your own combination! (60% vegetables, 40% fruits)

By the way, to help you keep track of your progress, I have also created a 4-week weight loss calendar for you to keep track of your progress. It's part of the bonus I included along with this ebook. Because I can't seem to format the schedule that fits all Kindle screens, you can download it and print it out for easier record-keeping :)

## Super Weight Loss Recipes

These are recipes which I've Googled from the Internet, tried them out myself, and proved to be EASY to do and effective in my weight loss goals.

What's great about my 4-Week Juicing for Weight Loss plan is that you have all the flexibility you can get while losing weight. I am not going to tie you down by saying that you MUST stick to Recipe A for week 1, and not be allowed to try another recipe which your tastebuds feel happier to have. This is also bearing in mind that you may not be able to obtain some of the ingredients as readily as others. While I try to keep the recipes as simple as possible, you also have the option of using recipes which require ingredients that you can easily buy from your farmer's market.

While I recommend you to go organic as much as possible, I know it may not be realistic as it can be very expensive. Opt to buy from your local farmer's market if possible. But remember, the purpose here to get you to incorporate Juicing into your lifestyle to lose weight. So unless going organic is something that really bothers you, I would prefer to do things one step at a time. :)

If you want more weight loss recipes, you can download them by visiting my page here.

**Super Weight Loss Juice**

According to SkinnyLimits, the secret ingredient to this recipe is the Cabbage! Throw in lemon and ginger to extra detoxifying effects to promote weight loss!

This recipe makes approximately 400-500ml of juice, perfect for breakfast or a mid-day juice.

3 Oranges (peeled) or 3 Apples
1/2 head of Young Cabbage
1/2 Lemon juice (or 1/2 lemon into your juicer)

1 Small Carrot

Thumb-sized piece of ginger

Ice (optional)

**ABC Detox Juice**

This is my favourite juice recipe and I just had to add it to this book! This is a great energising juice to have after a workout. Beet is also great for cleaning out your system!

1 Apple

1 Beet (around 2-3" in diameter)

1 Carrot or 1 Stalk or Celery

Note: If you haven't had beet before, it is good to start with half a beet, and eventually using a medium-sized beet.

**Fresh Start**

This juice recipe is great to start with for those who are trying to ease themselves into this whole juicing thing and they're not quite ready to drink those deep colored lookin' juices. If you need it even sweeter, just add another apple to it.

Don't think that just because it's said to be a "beginner juice" means it's not as good for you, this juice is great for you!

Ingredients
Apples - 2 medium (3" dia) 364g
Carrots - 3 medium 183g
Celery - 4 stalk, large (11"-12" long) 256g

**Weight Loss Juice #1**

**Makes about 14 ounces**

3 Carrots

1/2 Cucumber

1/2 Beet

1 Garlic Clove

2 Stalks Burdock root

## Weight Loss Juice #2

**Makes about 16 ounces**

3 Carrots

1/2 Cucumber

2 Celery Stalks

1/2 Bunch of Parsley

---

## Weight Loss Juice #3

**Makes about 16 ounces**

1 Medium Grapefruit

1 Medium Orange

1 Lemon

## Week 1

This is the week where you introduce yourself and your body to Juicing. Take it easy and remember, it's all about getting started on juicing, so there is no need to push yourself so hard.

During this week, try to eliminate other forms of liquids such as coffee, tea and milk. If you feel like you need that shot of espresso to prepare you for the rest of the day, have a juice FIRST, and then decide afterwards if you *really* need that coffee boost.

Drink enough water throughout the day to help flush your body of toxins. Some Juicers recommend infusing slices of lemon in your water or adding some pink Himalayan salt to alkalinise your water, but this is purely optional.

Pick one time of the day when having a juice is most convenient for you.

Because you are only consuming Juice once a day, pick out 2 recipes and alternate them. For example, you would have Weight Loss Juice Recipe #1 on Monday, #2 on Tuesday, and #1 on Wednesday again. At this point it is still alright to stick to 1 recipe since you are only drinking once a day, but I highly recommend some variations so to keep the novelty of it. :)

If you are using a centrifugal juicer, it is best to have your juice immediately after you prepare it. For many people, the most convenient time would either be in the morning before work/school, or at the end of the day.

If you are using a slow juicer and have prepared your juices in advance, this would be as simple as picking up your juice from refrigerator.

Prepare and consume your juice at the same time everyday during week 1. Here are some options:

- Have your juice immediately after you wake up
- Drink your juice 30 minutes before your meal
- Sip on your juice on your way to work (the same way some like to have their coffee on-the-go)

Remember that the goal is to make Juicing a part of your daily routine, so prepare and have it at the time which is most convenient to you. If you are usually rushing for work in the morning, then it will not be a good idea to juice in the morning as you are more likely to give up on it. Instead, opt for juicing at the end of the day where you can enjoy the preparation and enjoy the taste of your freshly-made juice.

Here is a Juicing plan for Week 1 which I recommend:

| Day | What to Juice? |
|---|---|
| 1 | Fresh Start |
| 2 | Fresh Start |
| 3 | ABC Juice |
| 4 | Fresh Start |
| 5 | Super Weight Loss Juice |
| 6 | Super Weight Loss Juice |
| 7 | Fresh Start |

## Week 2-3

Week 1 was really easy, wasn't it?

By now, you are already getting used to the idea of having Juice at least once a day, and you may experienced some weight loss! Congratulations!

If you haven't lost any weight, don't fret! Keep going and you will surely get the results you want.

Week 2 is about replacing one of your meals with juice, thereby increasing your intake of daily Juice.

During this week, you would have to use about 2-3 different recipes with varying ingredients, to ensure you're getting a variety of nutrients. With this in mind, you should be preparing about 32 ounces of juice per day. Since each of us have different perceptions of what is a "normal portion," I would recommend you to first consume 16 ounces of juice, wait it out, and if you feel hungry again, drink the rest of the juice you prepared for the day.

If after consuming your juice and you still feel hungry, consider making another glass of juice, or munching on some healthy snacks such as nuts.

Do not force-feed yourself the juice. If it is too much to drink in 1 sitting, sip on your juice over the hour. Taste the juice, think of how it feels like as the juice swirls around in your mouth. What ingredient stands out for you? Does the apple in the juice make it taste really savoury? Or does the cucumber feel refreshing? Do you feel the juice rushing through your system?

Write these feelings down, and they are going to help you figure out what juices appeal to you more, and become on your favourite list!

Remember: The goal of week 2 is to replace 1 meal with juice everyday.

Drink plenty of water throughout the rest of the day, and try to watch your food choices and portions for the rest of the day. For those who haven't lost any weight in week 1, this is the week you will start seeing the scale go down!

Again, there is flexibility in week 2, because you have more or less gotten used to the idea of juicing and making it part of your daily routine. You may wish to keep this up for the rest of your juicing for weight loss plan, until you hit your ideal weight. This plan of replacing 1 meal with juice each day will be sufficient to help you drop 1-4 pounds a week!

However, if after 2 weeks of replacing 1 meal a day with juice, you believe that you are ready to take things to the next level and possibly, challenge yourself, feel free to embark on week 3-4 of my plan!

| Day | Juice #1 to Replace Meal. | Juice #2 |
|---|---|---|
| 1 | Super Weight Loss Juice | Cucumber + Apple Juice |
| 2 | Beginner Green | Cucumber + Apple Juice |
| 3 | Weight Loss Juice #1 | ABC Juice |
| 4 | Weight Loss Juice #2 | Cucumber + Apple Juice |
| 5 | Beginner Green | ABC Juice |
| 6 | Super Weight Loss Juice | Cucumber + Apple Juice |
| 7 | Super Weight Loss Juice | Cucumber + Apple Juice |

Here are the additional recipes I introduced in Week 2:

**Cucumber + Apple Juice**

1 Cucumber
2 Apples
1/2 Lemon
Tiny piece of ginger to your liking (optional)

**Beginner Green**

1 Handful of Kale or Spinach
1 Cucumber
4 Sticks of Celery
2 Apples
1/2 Lemon
1" ginger piece

## Week 3-4

So, you're already set for the next phase of your weight loss plan, eh?

By this week you should be feeling awesome, becoming more awareness of your food choices and loving the Juicing lifestyle!

You would also be losing weight and maybe... you are excited about losing more weight quickly.

In this phase, you'll be replacing 2 meals a day with juice, while enjoying the texture of a solid meal once a day.

You don't have to feel bad if you can't seem to reach this phase. Remember I said in Week 2-3 that you can stick to replacing 1 meal a day and STILL be able to lose weight consistently each week.

For some of my friends, doing 2 meals of Juices a day didn't make much difference in weight loss as compared to only replacing 1 meal a day. On the other hand, I've also had friends who managed to fast-track their weight loss by replacing 2 meals a day. So this is really dependent on the individual body, your diet and activity level. See which one works best for you and your lifestyle.

If you have a hectic work schedule then you would probably find it easier to replace only 1 meal a day on weekdays, followed by replacing 2 meals a day over the weekend.

I do not intend to introduce a schedule for week 3-4 as this is the time for you to rotate the existing recipes as per my plan in week 2-3. Also, experiment with some Juicing recipes, see what you love best and feel free to use new recipes you find. To get ideas, you can also download my bonus to get more recipe ideas (www.JuicetoLoseWeight/Bonus)

**Keep these in mind when planning week 3-4 on your own:**

- Rotate the recipes and try not the have the same juice for more than 2 days in a row
- Try a variation of ingredients
- Experiment with different fruits to see which ones you like best

Remember that it is important that you incorporate Juicing into your lifestyle, so find an arrangement that allows you to stick to this habit. We are looking at a long-term goal of keeping the weight off forever, and you can only achieve it by making Juicing a part of your life!

Also, if you are going into Week 3-4, you may also want to allow yourself one cheat meal a week to indulge in foods you like (within reasonable limits), so that you won't feel deprived. I know I need my cheat meal because I can never bid farewell to my favourite pizza forever. :)

# Foods that Promote Weight Loss

Ready to take your weight loss plan to the next level? Incorporate these foods in your diet to enhance your weight loss plans:

**Ginger**

Used very often in Asian post-pregnancy diet, ginger helps to rid wind and remove toxins in the body. Use them in your cooking, juice them as we do in our recipes, or add a few slices into a glass of warm water or with your favourite tea to sip through the day.

**Brown Rice**

Brown rice is a low-energy-density food which means it is heavy and filling but low in calories. A serving of a half-cup has 1.7 grams of Resistant Starch which is a healthy carb that burns fat and boosts metabolism.

**Beans**

Beans are a good source of protein and fiber. They also contain Resistant Starch which helps boost metabolism and burn fat. Per half-cup of serving, garbanzo beans also called chickpeas only have more than 2 grams of Resistant Starch, white beans only contain 4 grams, while kidney beans only have nearly 2 grams.

**Quinoa**

Quinoa is a whole grain which is diet-friendly and is rich in hunger-fighting protein. You stay full longer and avoid overeating at meals.

**Oats**

Oats are rich in fiber and a serving can make you feel full throughout the day. Oats also contain Resistant Starch.

**Salmon**

Salmon is a lean source of protein which can make you feel full minus the fat.

**Wine**

The antioxidant called resveratrol found in grape skin stops the storage of fat. Based on studies, moderate wine drinkers have less belly fat than the liquor drinkers.

**Nuts**

Take a handful of peanuts, almonds, pecans, or walnuts for a snack and you eat less at later meals.

**Lentils**

Lentils are another source of fiber and protein. A half-cup has 3.4 grams of Resistant Starch.

**Apple**

Apples contain fiber and can blunt the appetite. Chewing on the crunchy apple sends signal to the brain that you have eaten something substantial.

**Grapefruit**

Researchers found that when obese people ate half a grapefruit before each meal, they lost an average of 3.5 pounds over 12 weeks. Though it does not have proven fat-burning properties, it may have helped people feel full much longer.

**Blueberries**

Aside from being known for its anti-aging properties, blackberries only have 80 calories per one cup serving and contain 4 grams of fiber which can help you feel full.

**Avocados**

Avocados contain oleic acid which can help your body suppress hunger. A quarter or half of an avocado may help melt your belly fat away. It is also packed with fiber and protein.

**Bananas**

A medium-size and slightly green banana can fill you up and boost your metabolism since it contains 12.5 grams of Resistant Starch. A ripe banana contains 5 grams Resistant Starch.

**Drinks that help the body detox**

It is best to combine a reduced-calorie diet with beverages that detoxify the body, making you feel and look much more fit and healthier. Below are some of the recommended health drinks for those who are trying to lose weight:

**Green Tea**

Green tea has gained popularity because of its supposed benefits for weight loss. Green tea is high in antioxidants which can fight disease and is also very good for the liver, the body's main detox organ.

**Lemon Water**

Starting your day with a cup of hot lemon water can aid your body in burning more fat. It helps the body detox and aid in digestion. Drink hot lemon water after you wake up each morning for its digestive-cleansing benefits.

**Green Juice**

With a juicer, make a green juice from ingredients with naturally detoxifying properties such as spinach, lemon, watercress, and ginger.

**Water**

Water keeps the body properly hydrated, and with the right water levels, the liver and other detox organs in the body will function well.

## Final Words on Juicing to Lose Weight

Okay! I am feeling very nervous about this, but... I'm now setting you free!

Yes, freedom to experiment with Juice recipes and to find an arrangement that works best for you to make Juicing a part of your life.

Remember, I'm here for you, so whenever you have any questions about Juicing to Lose Weight, you can also drop me an email to juicetoloseweight@gmail.com

Don't forget to claim your BONUS by heading to JuicetoLoseWeight.com where I share more Juice recipes that you can use. You don't necessarily have to stick to the Weight Loss recipes I share here, because as long as you make Juicing a part of your daily life, you will surely be able to get the weight loss results you want, and keep them permanent.

Could you also do me a favour? If you enjoyed this book, please leave a review on Amazon! I'll be updating the book with new information as I go along, so your feedback is valuable to me!

Cheers to your juicing success!

## Troubleshooting

**"Yuck! The Juice tastes too bitter!"**

Simple problem to solve. Simply add more fruits to the recipe to combat the undesirable taste. If the recipe called for 3 apples, increase it to 1-2 more apples to sweeten up the taste!

**"I'm sick of using Kale over and over again."**

The beauty of Juicing is that you don't have to stick to a rigid recipe. You can rotate your green leafy vegetables. If you've been having too much Kale, switch to Spinach instead.

**"I'm still hungry even after drinking so much juice!"**

Don't feel guilty if you need to eat to feel satisfied. Try to drink a glass of water and wait for another 30 minutes before deciding if you're really hungry.

Ask yourself, are you really hungry or is it just you craving for some food? If you are thinking of a specific food in mind (like a burger), then it is most likely just a craving and not hunger. If you feel you must eat, then go ahead and don't feel bad about. Instead, aim to gradually decrease the food you eat after juicing, until you are able to successfully replace 1 meal with Juice.

Have more troubleshooting questions? Send me an email to juicetoloseweight@gmail.com

**Copyright Information and Disclaimer**



This eBook is an information product on Juicing to Lose Weight. By reading this eBook you agree to the following terms:

The content in this eBook is not a substitute for direct, personal or professional medical advice or diagnosis. None of the treatments, remedies, and/or recommendations should be followed without consulting with a professionally trained therapist or the mutual consent of both parties.

There may be risks associated with actively practicing the activities and/or advice mentioned in this book for people with poor health, or with pre-existing physical/mental mention or physical/mental health conditions. Following the advice given in this eBook is done on your own free will and accord.

Under no circumstances, including, but no limited to, negligence, shall the copyright owner, be liable for any special or consequential damages, so the above limitation or exclusion may not apply to you.

In no event shall the copyright holder's total liability to you for all damages, losses and causes of action exceed the amount paid by you, if any, for this book.

You agree to hold the owner(s) of this eBook, the agents, co-authors, contributors, affiliates and employees harmless from any and all liability for all claims for damages due to injuries, including attorney fees and costs incurred by you or caused to third parties by you, arising out of the use and advice of this eBook.

Fact and information are believed to be accurate at the time that this book was written. All data provided in this eBook is to be used for information purposes only.

Information provided is not all-inclusive and is limited to information made available and such information should not be relied upon as all-inclusive or accurate.

IF YOU DO NOT AGREE WITH THESE TERMS AND CONDITIONS, DO NOT CONTINUE TO READ THIS EBOOK. YOUR USE OF THIS EBOOK, PRODUCTS, SERVICES AND ANY PARTICIPATION OF THE ACTIVITIES MENTIONED IN THIS EBOOK MEANS THAT YOU ARE AGREEING TO BE LEGALLY BOUND BY THESE TERMS.

17983578R00037

Printed in Great Britain
by Amazon